BUSY PLACES

Hospital

Carol Watson

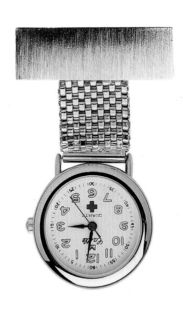

W

FRANKLIN WATTS

NEW YORK • LONDON • SYDNEY

It's morning at the hospital.
All over the building people
are busy doing their jobs
and helping sick people to get well.

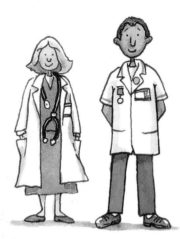

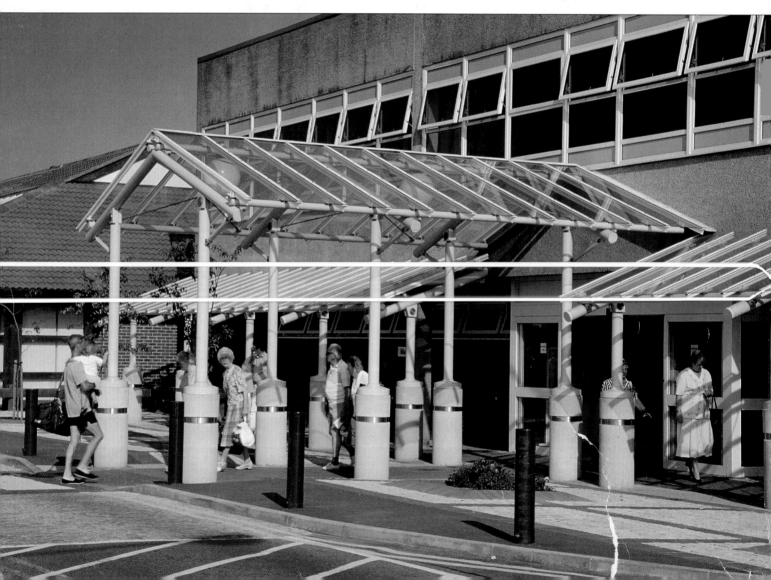

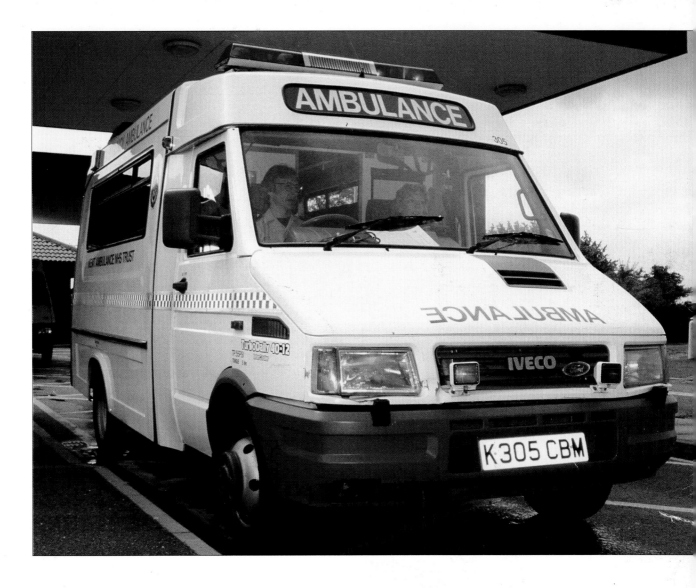

Outside the hospital the ambulance teams
wait to see where they are needed.
They go to collect people who have
had accidents or are seriously ill.

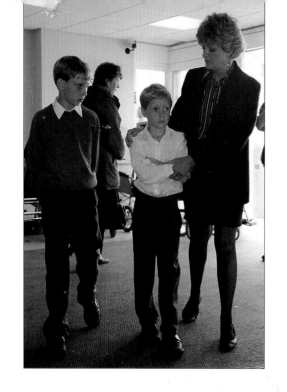

Inside the hospital Mrs Crux has arrived with her two sons. Justin has fallen off his bicycle and hurt his arm.

The receptionist asks them to wait in the Accident and Emergency Department.

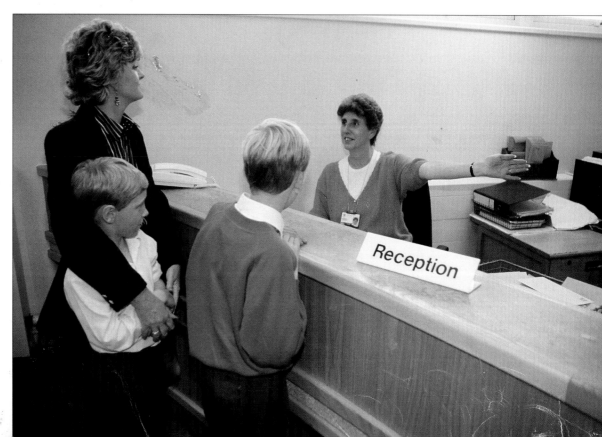

4

Soon it is Justin's turn to see Doctor Roberts.
She gently examines his arm.
"Where exactly does it hurt?" the doctor asks him.
Justin points to the spot.

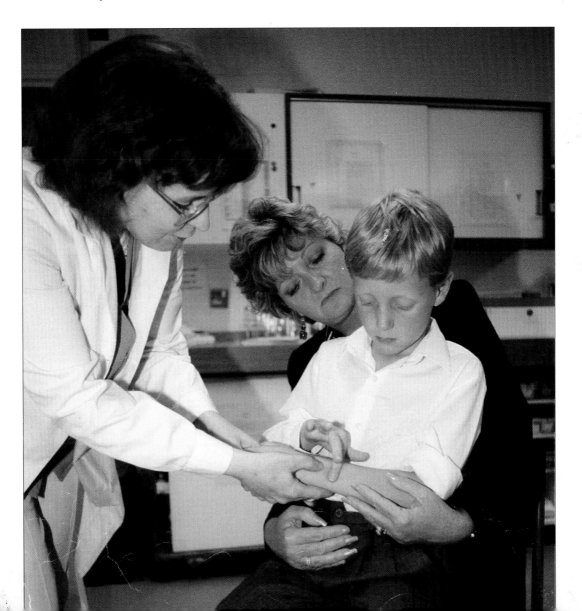

Doctor Roberts sends Justin for an X-ray.
Then she shows it to the two boys.
"The X-ray shows that you have broken your wrist,"
the doctor explains.

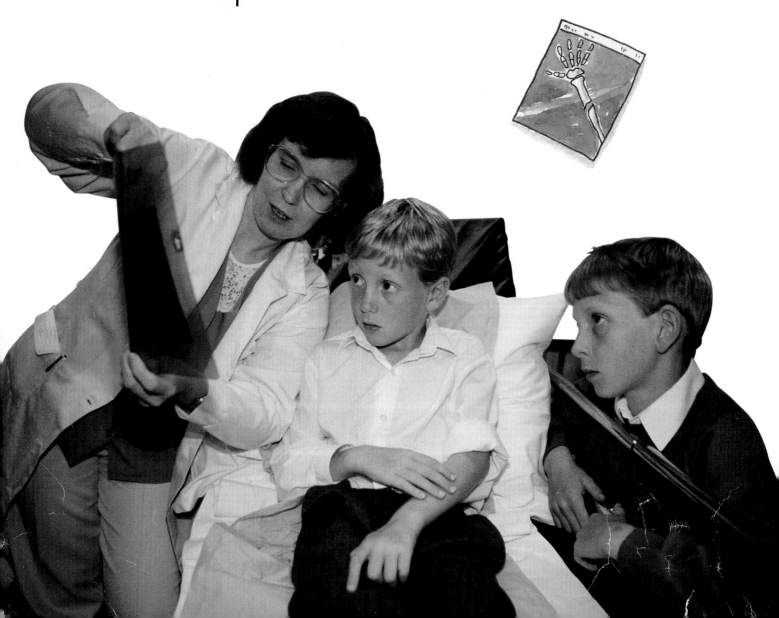

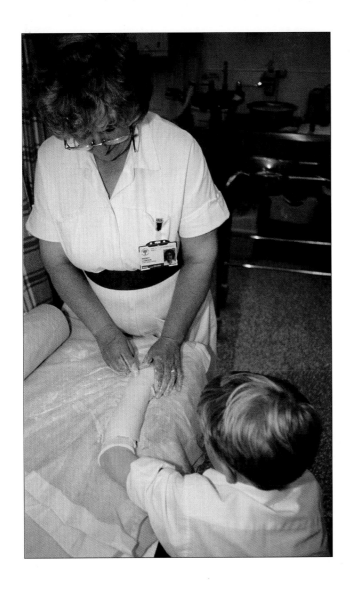

The Staff Nurse puts his arm in plaster. "That will keep your arm in one position," she says. "Then the bone will heal properly."

Justin goes to the Fracture Clinic.

Nurses wear their watches pinned onto their uniform. Their watches hang upside down. Can you think why?

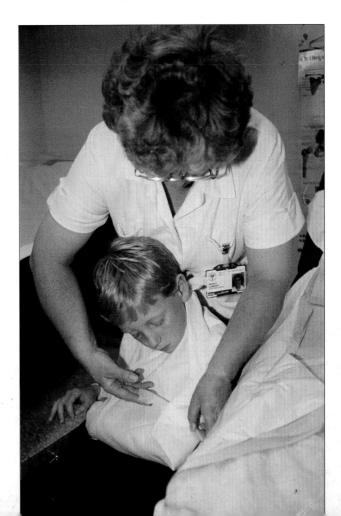

In the Physiotherapy
Department, patients
are doing exercises
to help parts of their bodies
that are stiff or painful.

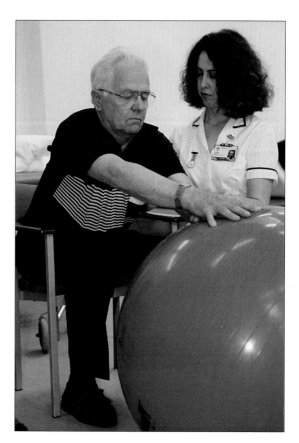

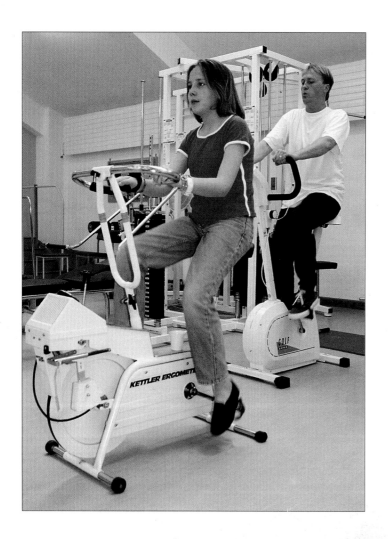

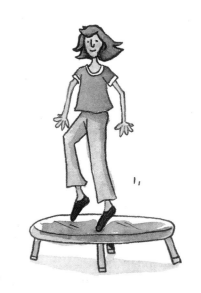

Some of the patients are treated as they float in a large pool of warm water. "Can you move your legs, Mrs Jones?" asks one of the physiotherapists.

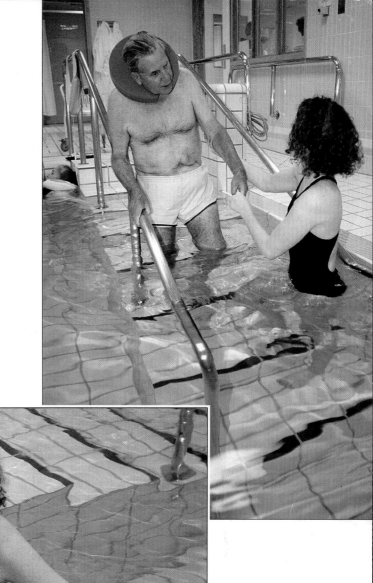

On Padua Ward, the Sister and Nurse are discussing the patients in their care.
"Tim is having his operation this afternoon," says Sister Culleton.

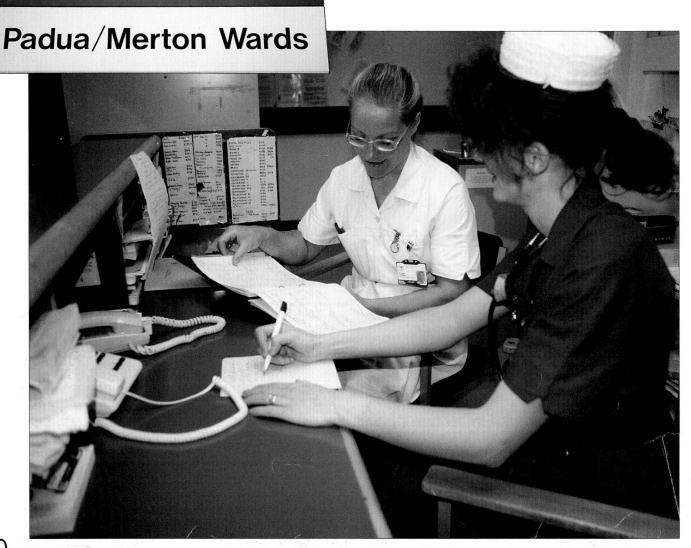

Padua/Merton Wards

The Sister talks to Tim about
what is going to happen to him.
"Don't worry," she says.
"You'll soon be feeling much better."

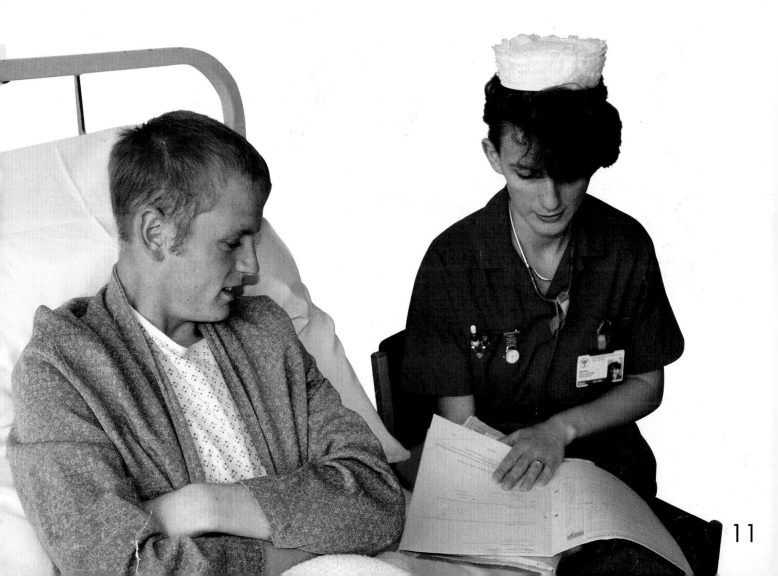

When it is time for Tim's operation a porter pushes him on a trolley towards the operating theatre. They go up in a lift.

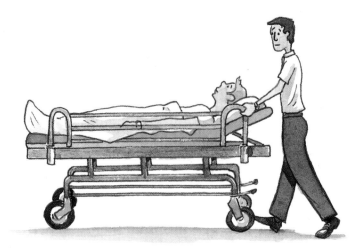

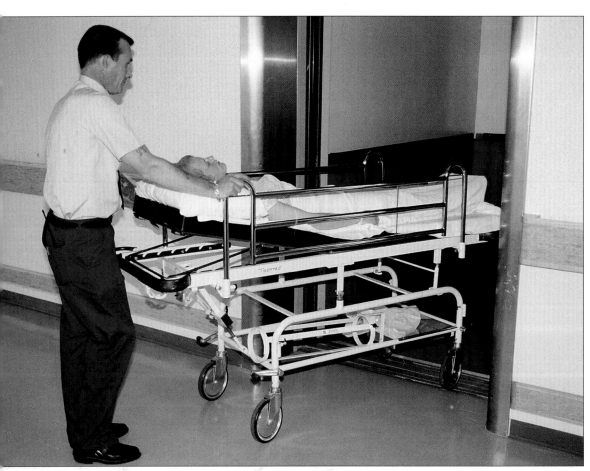

Meanwhile, in another operating theatre a patient is already on the operating table. The surgeon and her team prepare for work.

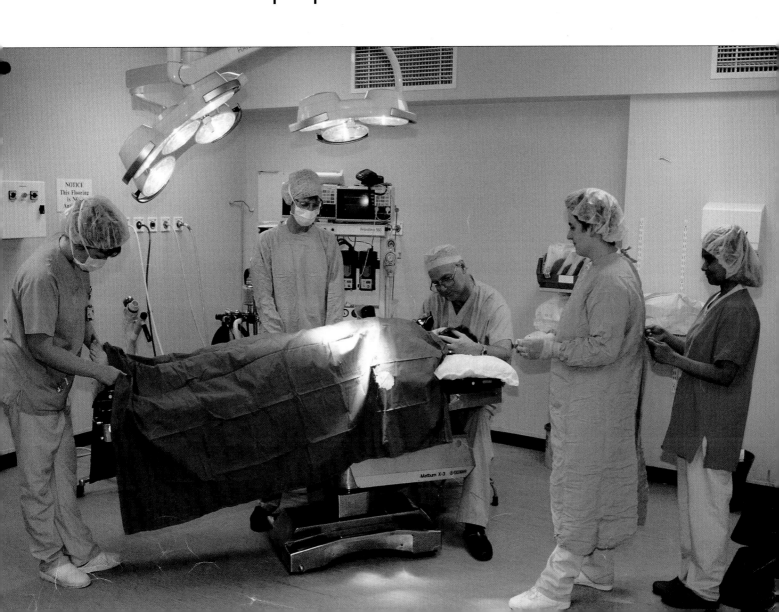

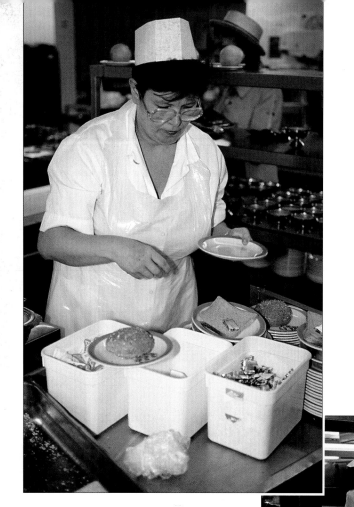

Downstairs in the
hospital kitchen
the catering staff
are getting lunch ready.
"It's 12.30," says
the Supervisor.
"We can start serving
the meals now."

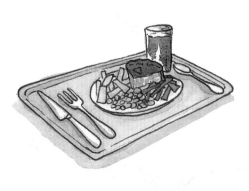

14

A porter takes the hot meals from the kitchen to the patients on the wards.

In the canteen some of the hospital staff eat together and relax.

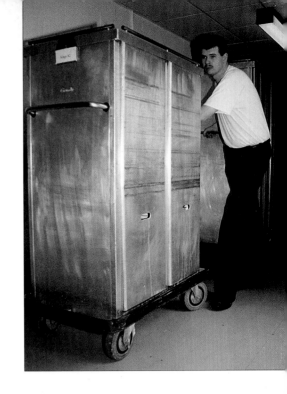

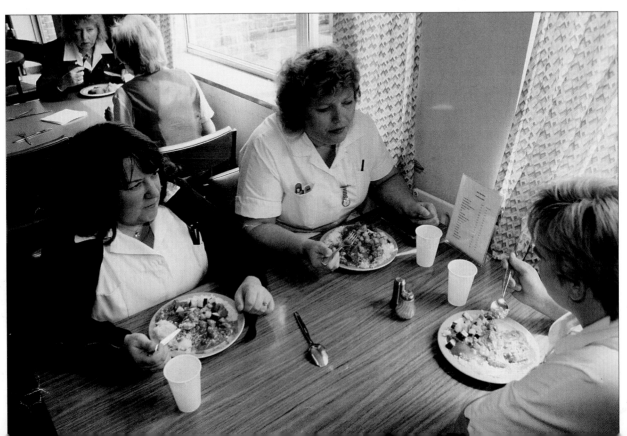

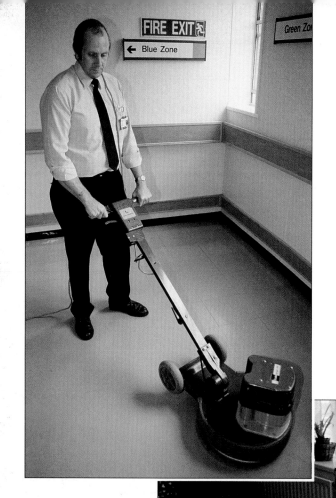

In other parts of the hospital
people are hard at work.
A cleaner uses a machine
to polish the floors.

In the office the secretaries
are busy typing letters and
keeping records.

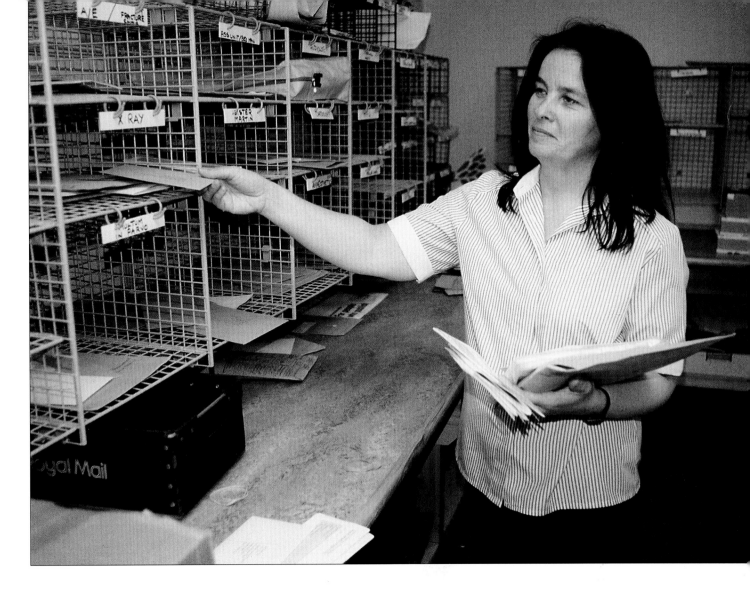

In the post room a large sack of mail has arrived.
"There's a lot of post for the
X-Ray Department," Sue says to herself
as she sorts the letters.

The Pharmacy Department is where
the medicines and pills are kept.
The Pharmacists supply them
to all the patients in the hospital.

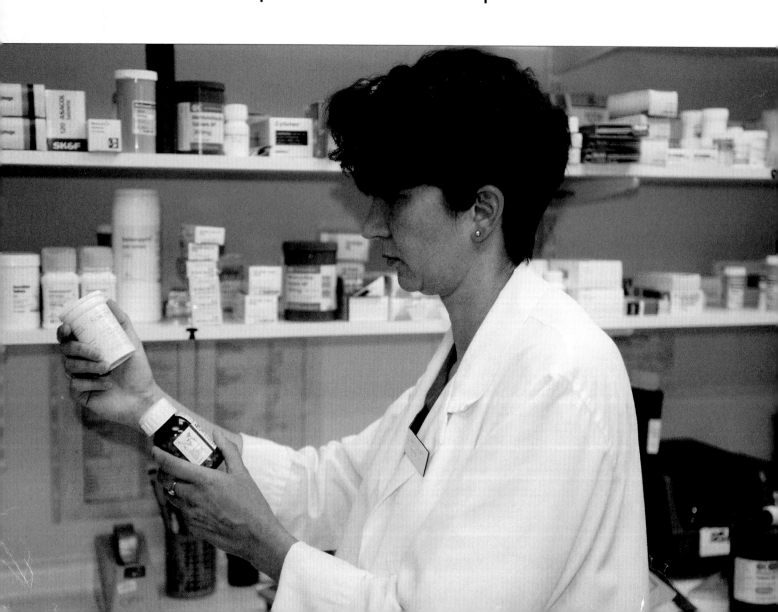

Chris gives some tablets to a patient who has visited one of the clinics. "Take one of these three times a day after meals," he tells her.

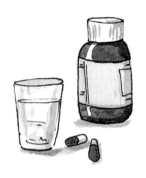

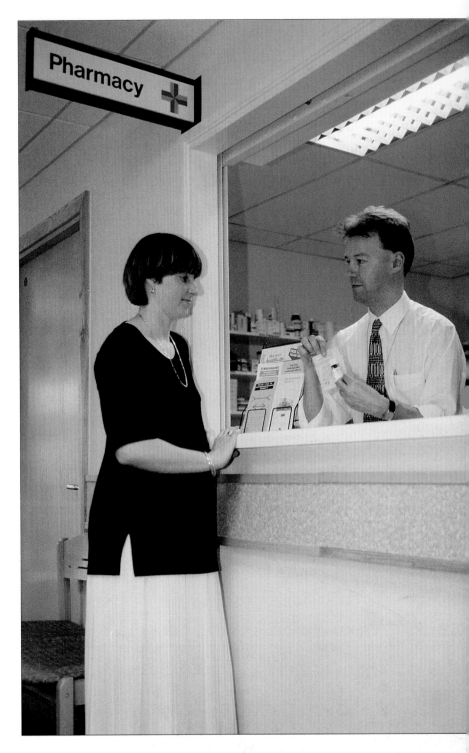

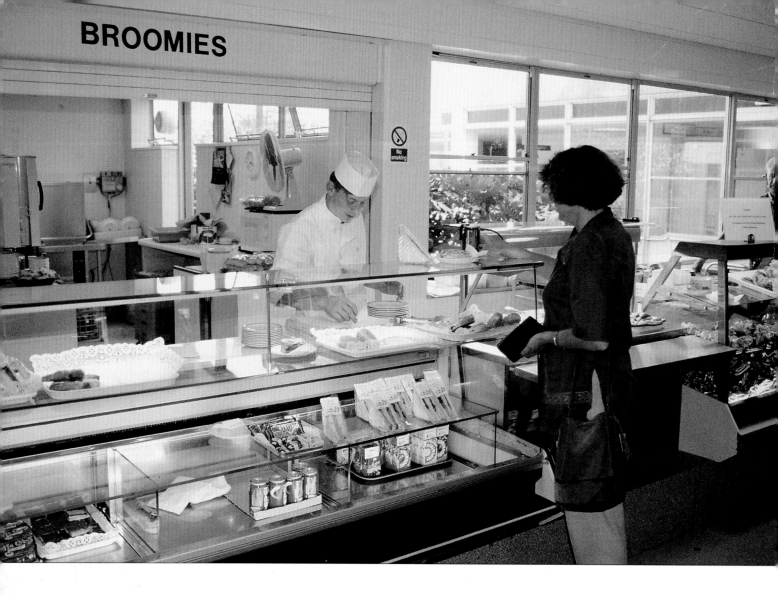

In the coffee shop staff are busy serving customers.
Clare has arrived at the hospital to visit Tim.
"Can I have some sandwiches and
a cake, please?" she asks.

After her snack Clare goes to
the hospital flower shop.
She buys a bunch of flowers
for Tim. "That will be four pounds,
please," says the florist.

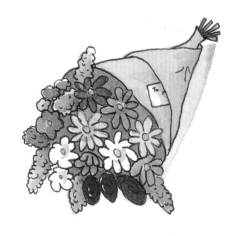

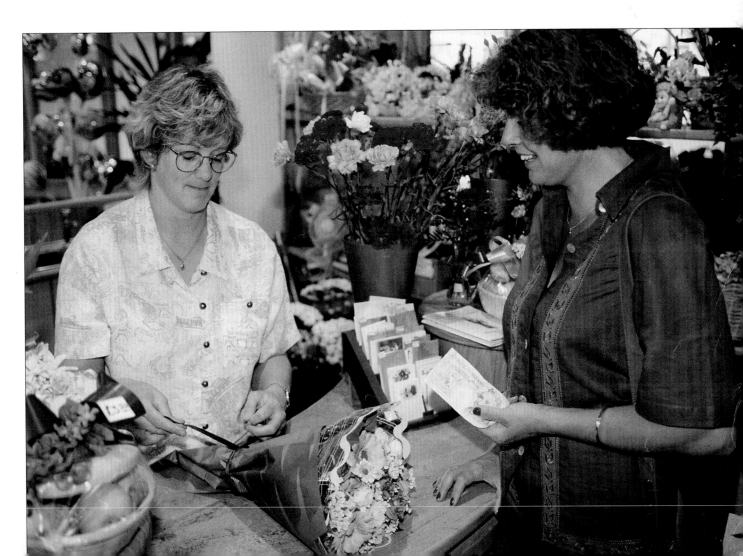

It's visiting time on Padua Ward.
Tim is back in his bed after his operation.
"How are you feeling?" asks Clare.
"I'm fine," he says. "Everyone here
has looked after me very well."

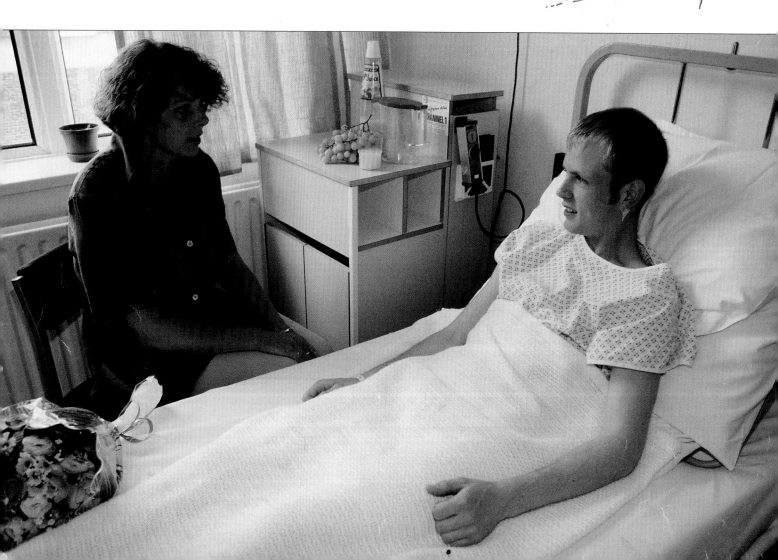

Care and safety in a hospital

When you are in a busy hospital it is important to make sure that you and others keep safe.

Try to remember some of these tips:

1. Always stay well away from hospital machines and never touch any knobs or switches.

2. Don't run around the wards or corridors.

3. Move out of the way if you see a porter pushing a trolley or any other equipment.

4. If you are a patient do not eat or drink anything unless the nurse says that you can.

5. If you are a visitor always stay close to your parent or friend.

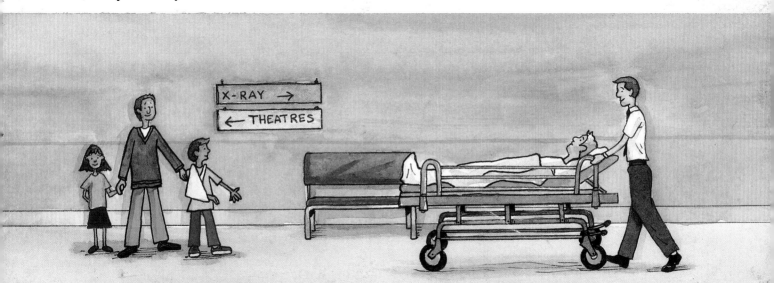

Index

© 1998 Franklin Watts
96 Leonard Street
London
EC2A 4RH

Franklin Watts Australia
14 Mars Road
Lane Cove
NSW 2066

ISBN 0 7496 2978 9

Dewey Decimal Classification Number
610

A CIP catalogue record for this book is
available from the British Library

Printed in Hong Kong

Editor: Samantha Armstrong
Designer: Kirstie Billingham
Photographer: Steve Shott
Illustrations: Richard Morgan

With thanks to Kay Curtis and all the
staff at The William Harvey Hospital,
South Kent Hospitals NHS Trust,
Justin and Oliver Crux and Tim Purner.

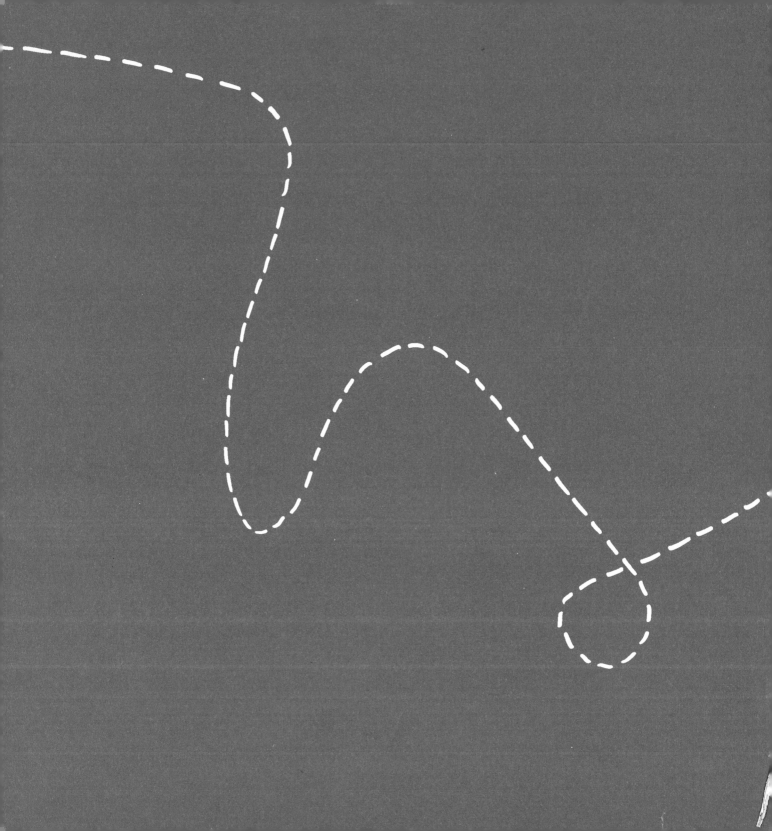